LET FOOD BE YOUR MEDICINE

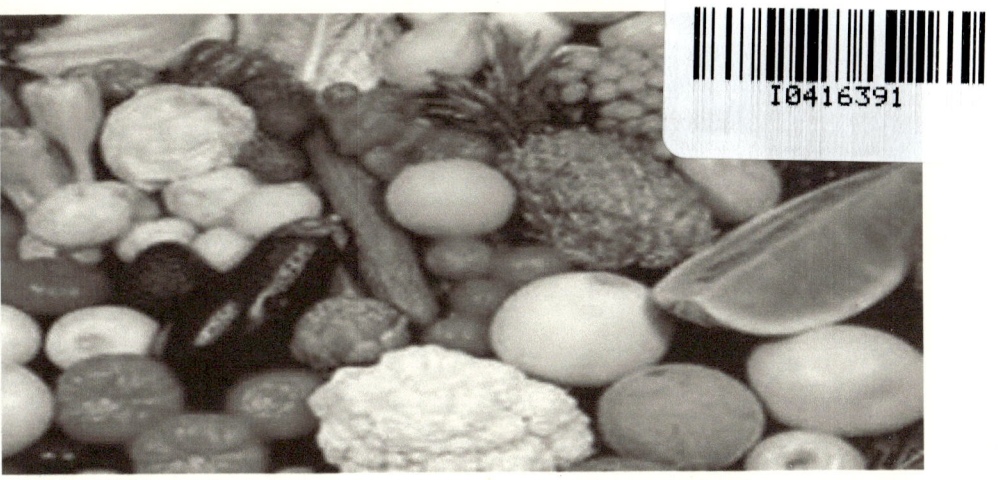

Contents

Forward Notes

I always have to ascribe glory and praise to Almighty God. He is the one who continues to give me new ideas, concepts and insight for venturing into deeper waters. I am not afraid to launch out or afraid to make mistakes. I put all of my trust in the true and living God and He always makes away for me to succeed.

For the Spirit God gave us does not make us timid, but gives us power, love and self-discipline. 2 Timothy 1:7. Fear is the enemy of entrepreneurship. God wants us to step out in faith with the power he gives us to pursue our ideas, not only in ministry but in business also.

I can publicly say that what I know today about health issues I didn't know many years ago. And I can also say without any apology that I am never ashamed of my age. Today I feel more alert, energized and enthusiastic than I did 30 years ago, all because I decided to change my life style and eating habits.

1 Corinthian 10:31 says "So, whether you eat or drink, or whatever you do, do all to the glory of God in your body". I don't mind telling people how old I am because I feel ageless! Thanks for your support in purchasing my books.

Bishop Dr. Juliette D. Fagan, Prof Natural Health Practitioner, Clinical Colon Therapist

Introduction

Natural health cures is a constructive method of treatment which aims at removing the basic cause of disease through the rational use of the elements freely available in nature itself. With all of the pollution in the environment none of us can escape the attacks. I will do my endeavor best to share some of the things I have studied and learnt over the years as it pertains to allopathic or conventional medicine and naturopathic or alternative medicine.

Although the term 'naturopathy' is of relatively recent origin, the philosophical basis and several of the methods of natural remedies and treatments are ancient. It was practiced in ancient Egypt, Greece and Rome. Hippocrates, the father of medicine (460-357 B.C.) strongly advocated natural cures and that food should be our medicine. After training and working as a nurse for several years I decided to become a naturopathic practitioner.

After studying alternative medicine I found out that the whole mass of knowledge about natural cures done over the years was later collected under one name, Naturopathy. The credit for the name Naturopathy goes to Dr. Benedict Lust (1872 - 1945), and hence he is called the Father of Naturopathy. Natural cures and remedies is based on the realization that man was created by God and is born healthy and strong and that he can stay as such if he lives in accordance with the laws of nature. Even if one is born with some inherited affliction, the individual can eliminate it by putting to the best use the natural agents of healing. Fresh air, sunshine, a proper diet, exercise, relaxation, constructive thinking, the right mental attitude, along with prayer, fasting and faith in supernatural healing, all play their part in keeping a sound mind in a sound body.

Natural health practitioners believe that disease is an abnormal condition of the body resulting from the violation of the natural laws of nature. Every such violation has repercussions on the human system in the shape of lowered vitality, irregularities of the blood, lymph, colon and the accumulation of waste matter and toxins.

Thus, through a faulty diet and poor elimination of waste it is not the digestive system alone which is adversely affected. When toxins accumulate, other organs such as the bowels, kidneys, skin and lungs are overworked and cannot get rid of these harmful substances as quickly as they are produced. Besides this, mental and emotional disturbances cause imbalances of the human electric field within which cell metabolism takes place, producing toxins. When the cellular level is undisturbed and nourished, disease-causing germs can live in it without multiplying or producing toxins. It is only when it is disturbed or when the blood is polluted with toxic waste that the germs multiply and become harmful.

I am not a professional writer but I have a desire to educate all who are willing to learn and make adjustments in their daily walks of life. I know as I practice I will become more perfect. Thanks for your patience and understanding and I know you will learn something from what I have written in this and my other books.

Chapter 1

Principles and Practice of Natural remedies

The first and most basic principle of nature cures (natural health) is that all forms of disease are due to the same cause, namely, the accumulations of waste materials and bodily waste in the system. These waste materials in the healthy individual are removed from the system through the organs of elimination. But in the diseased person, they are steadily piling up in the body through years of faulty eating habits, improper care of the body and habits contributing to stress and nervous exhaustion such as worry, overwork, alcohol, smoking and excesses of all kinds. It follows from this basic principle that the only way to cure diseases naturally is to employ methods which will enable the system to throw off and get rid of these toxic accumulations. All natural health treatments are actually directed towards this end.

The second basic principle of nature cures is that all acute (short term) diseases such as fevers, colds, inflammations, digestive disturbances and skin eruptions are nothing more than self-initiated efforts on the part of the body to throw off the accumulated waste materials and that all chronic diseases such as heart disease, diabetes, multiple sclerosis, lupus, rheumatism, asthma, kidney disorders, are the results of continued suppression of the acute diseases through harmful methods such as drugs, vaccines, narcotics, artificial energy stimulants. Mostly all diseases are autoimmune diseases caused by the body attacking itself.

The third principle of nature or natural cures is that the body was created by God to heal itself and contains an elaborate healing mechanism which has the power to bring about a return to normal condition of health, provided right methods are employed to enable it to do so. In other words, the power to cure disease lies within the body itself and not in the hands of others. I am in no way advocating sick persons must not go to medical doctors, I am a trained natural health practitioner and specializes in education about the benefits of natural cures, remedies and the benefit of organic food. Please see your medical doctor and follow his or her instructions and never stop taking your medication as prescribed by your doctor.

Chapter 2

Natural Remedies vs Modern System

Personally I don't think that anything I am saying here is at all foreign to you my readers. The modern or conventional medical system treats the symptoms and suppresses the disease but does very little to ascertain the real root cause. Toxic drugs which may suppress or relieve some ailments usually all have harmful side-effects on the organs. Over the years of studying and doing my own research I must admit that most drugs usually hinder the self-healing efforts of the body and make recovery more difficult and can even take longer.

According to the late Sir William Osler of Ontario Canada, an eminent physician and surgeon, when drugs are used, the patient has to recover twice - once from the illness, and once from the drug. It's time for the truth to be told, that drugs cannot cure diseases; the disease might be halted but it continues. It is only its pattern that changes. Drugs also produce dietary deficiencies by destroying nutrients in some instances, by using them up, and preventing their absorption. Moreover, the toxicity that drugs produce at a time when the body is least capable of coping with it.

The power to restore health thus lies not in drugs alone, but in nature itself. The approach of modern system is more on combative lines after the disease has set in, whereas natural health practices lays greater emphasis on preventive method and measures to attain and maintain health and prevent disease. The modern medical system treats each disease as a separate entity, requiring specific

9

drug for its cure, whereas naturopathy treats the organism as a whole and seeks to restore harmony to the whole of the patient's being.

Chapter 3

Methods of Natural Health

The nature cure system aims at the readjustment of the human system from abnormal to normal conditions and functions, and adopts methods of cure which are in conformity with the constructive principles of nature itself. Proper administered natural health methods remove from the system the accumulation of toxic matter and poisons without in any way injuring the vital organs of the body. They also stimulate the organs of elimination and purification to better functioning.

To rid the body of disease, the first and foremost requirement is to regulate the diet. To get rid of accumulated toxins and restore the equilibrium of the system, it is desirable to completely exclude acid-forming foods, including proteins, starches and fats, for a week or more and to confine the diet to fresh fruits which will disinfect the stomach and alimentary canal.

If the body is overloaded with morbid matter, as in acute disease, a complete fast for a few days may be necessary for the elimination of toxins. Fruit juice may, however, be taken during a health related fast. A simple rule is: do not eat when you are sick, stick to a light diet of fresh fruits. Wait for the return of the usual healthy appetite. Loss of appetite is Nature's warning that no burden should be placed on the digestive organs. Let me make it clear that this book is not based on the way us Christians do a spiritual fast, where abstain from food or hold a partial fast. I will be discussing the benefits of fasting in general.

Alkaline foods such as raw vegetables and sprouted whole grain cereals may be added after a week of a fruits-only diet. Another important factor in the cure of diseases by natural methods is to stimulate the vitality of the body. This can be achieved by using water in various ways and at varying temperatures in the form of packs or baths. The application of cold water, especially to the abdomen, the seat of most diseases, and to the sexual organs, through a cold sitting (hip) bath immediately lowers body heat and stimulates the nervous system.

In the form of wet packs, hydro (water) therapy offers a simple natural method of lowering fevers and reducing pain and inflammation without any harmful side-effects. Warm water applications, on the other hand, are relaxing. Other natural methods useful in the cure of diseases are fresh air, regular sun shine, exercise, therapeutic massages and having a positive mind are all good physically, spiritually, emotionally and mentally.

Fresh air and the sun revive dead skin and help maintain it in a normal condition. Exercise, no matter how small helps to promote inner health and harmony and helps eliminate all tension: physically, mentally and emotionally. Massage tones up the nervous system and quickens blood circulation and the metabolic process. Thus a well-balanced diet, sufficient physical exercise, fresh air, plenty of sunlight, pure drinking water, cleanliness, adequate rest, right mental attitude and getting rid of all resentment, worries, fear, doubt, anger and unforgiveness can also ensure proper health and prevent disease. Remember nature's food still has the ability to heal the body.

Chapter 4

Obesity

Obesity may be described as a bodily condition characterized by excessive deposition or storage of fat in adipose tissue. It usually results from consumption of food in excess of physiological needs. Obesity is common among people in Western countries and among the higher income groups and developing countries. Obesity can occur at any age in either sex. Its incidence is higher in persons who consume more food and lead sedentary lives.

Among women, obesity is liable to occur after pregnancy and during menopause. A woman usually gains weight during pregnancy. Part of this is an increase in the adipose tissue which serves as a store against the demands of lactation. Many women gain more and retain part of this weight. They become progressively obese with each succeeding child if they do not exercise and have self-control over their eating habits. Obesity is a serious health hazard as the extra fats puts a strain on the heart, kidneys and liver as well as the large weight-bearing joints such as the hips, knees and ankles, which ultimately shortens the life span.

It has been truly said, 'the longer the belt, the short the life' Over weight persons are susceptible to several diseases like coronary thrombosis, heart failure, high blood pressure, diabetes, arthritis, gout, liver, gall-bladder and reproductive organ disorders.

Chief Cause of Obesity

The chief cause of obesity, most often, is overeating - that is, the intake of calories beyond the body's energy requirement. Some people are habituated to eating too much while others may be in the habit of consuming high-calorie junk foods. These people gain weight continuously as they fail to adjust their appetite to reduce energy requirements. There has, in recent times, been an increase in awareness of psychological aspects of obesity. Persons who are generally bored , unhappy, lonely, depressed or feel unloved, those who are discontented with their family members, spouse, social or financial standing usually tend to overeat as eating is a pleasure and solace to them. Obesity is sometimes also the result of disturbances of the thyroid or pituitary glands. But glandular disorders account for only about two per cent of the total incidence of obesity. In such persons, the basal metabolism rate is low and they keep gaining weight unless they take a low-calorie diet, exercise and discipline themselves.

Chapter 5

Plan of Action

A suitably planned course of dietetic treatment, in conjunction with suitable exercise and other measures for promoting elimination is the only scientific way of dealing with obesity and weight lost. The chief consideration in all of this should be the balanced selection of foods which provide the maximum essential nutrients with the least number of calories. To begin with, the individual should undertake a juice fast for seven to ten days. Juices of lemon, grape fruit, orange, pineapple, cabbage and celery, may be taken during this period.

Long juice fast should only be undertaken under expert guidance and supervision. In the alternative, short juice fasts should be repeated at regular intervals of two months or so till the desired reduction in weight is achieved. Let emphasis again, losing weight requires discipline.

First things first, follow these four rules: 1.Chew your food to a pulp or milky liquid until it practically swallows itself. 2. Never eat until you are really hungry. 3 Enjoy every bite of your food until it is swallowed. 4 Do not eat when tired, angry, in a rush or worried.

I also understand that ingestion of small amounts of natural honey is an excellent home remedy for obesity. It mobilizes the extra deposited fat in the body and puts it into circulation which is utilized as energy for normal functions. I suggest you start with a small quantity of about taken with hot water. The dose can be gradually increased.

A natural weight loss program is fasting 7-21 days (even up to 30 days) on honey - lemon juice and water. This is highly beneficial in the treatment of obesity without the loss of energy and appetite. In this mode of treatment, one spoon of fresh honey should be mixed with a juice of half a lemon or lime in a glass of

lukewarm water and taken at regularly intervals. Stay away from TV or commercial diet fads. Take your time and regain your desired body weight.

Another effective remedy for obesity is an exclusive lemon juice diet. Leeroy and I have done this fast several times, also some of the brethren at church with great results. Some call it the master cleanse and some the lemon diet.

On the first day you should have nothing but plenty of water. On the second day juice of three lemons mixed with equal amount of water. One lemon should be subsequently increased each day until the juice of 12 lemons is consumed per day. Then the number of lemons should be decreased in the same order until three lemons are taken in a day. Remember you might feel weak and hungry on the first two days, but afterwards the condition will subside by itself. Again I say, take your time.

Cabbage is also considered to be an effective home remedy for obesity. Recent research has discovered in cabbage is a valuable content which inhibits the conversion of sugar and other carbohydrates into fat. Hence, fresh cabbage juice is of great value in weight reduction. Also a helping of cabbage salad would be the simplest way to stay slim, but raw cabbage is said to cause bloating so monitor your body. I recommend the cabbage juice.

Cabbage is found to possess the maximum biological value with minimum calorific value. Moreover, it gives a lasting feeling of fullness in the stomach and is easily digestible. Along with dietetic treatment, one should always adopt all other natural methods of reducing weight. Exercise is an important part of weight reduction plan and there is no short cut. It helps to use up calories stored in body fat and relieves tension, besides toning up the muscles of the body. Walking is the best exercise to begin with and may be followed by aerobics. Not only does exercise break up or re-distribute fatty deposits and help slimming, but it also strengthen the flabby areas, am sure some of you know exactly what am talking about. You always want to get to a measure which brings on excessive perspiration. Excess sweating also helps to reduce weight. Above all, obese persons should make every effort to avoid the feeling of low self-esteem and negative emotions such as anxiety, fear, hostility and insecurity. You are not a mistake, God created you for a purpose. You have to want a change in your life.

Chapter 6

The Power of Fasting

Fasting refers to complete abstinence from food for a short or long period for a specific purpose. The word is derived from the old English, 'faestan' which means to fast, observe, be strict, abstinence from food. Fasting is nature's oldest, most effective and yet least expensive method of treating disease naturally and weight lost. The common cause of all diseases is the accumulation of waste and poisonous matter in the body which results from overeating. Majority of persons eat too much and follow sedentary occupations which do not permit sufficient and proper exercise for utilization of this large quantity of food. This surplus overburdens the digestive and assimilative organs and clogs up the system with impurities or poisons.

Digestion and elimination become slow and the functional activity of the whole system gets deranged. The onset of disease is merely the process of ridding the system of these impurities. Every disease can be healed by only one remedy - by doing just the opposite of what causes it, that is, by reducing the food intake and fasting. By depriving the body of food for a time the organs of elimination such as the bowels, kidneys, skin and lungs are given opportunity to expel accumulated waste from the system. Thus, fasting is merely the process of purification and an effective and quick method of cleansing. Fasting assists nature in its continuous effort to expel foreign matter and disease producing waste products from the body, thereby correcting the faults of improper diet. It also leads to regeneration of the blood as well as the repair and regeneration of the various cells and tissues of the body.

The duration of the fast depends upon the age of the individual, the nature of the disease and the amount and type of drugs previously used. The duration is important, because long periods of fasting can be dangerous if undertaken without competent professional guidance. It is, therefore, advisable to undertake a series of short fasts of two to three days and gradually increase the duration of each succeeding fast by a day or so. The period, however, should not exceed a week of total fasting at a time. This will enable the chronically sick body to gradually and slowly eliminate toxic waste matter without seriously affecting the natural functioning of the body. A correct mode of living and a balanced diet after the fast will restore vigor and vitality to the individual. Fasting is highly beneficial in practically all kinds of stomach and intestinal disorders and in serious conditions of the kidneys and liver.

It is a miracle cure for eczema and other skin diseases and offers the only hope of permanent cure in many cases. The various nervous disorders also respond favorably to this mode of natural treatment. Fasting should, however, not be done in all illness.

Incases of diabetes, advanced stages of tuberculosis, and extreme cases of neurasthenia (weakening of nerves), Very long fasts can be harmful in some instances. In most cases, however, no harm will accrue to fasting, provided persons take rest, and are under proper professional care and supervision.

Chapter 7

Fasting Methods

The best, safest and most effective method of fasting is juice fasting. Although the old classic form of fasting especially in the church was and is still practiced, is what we call a pure water fast, done more on a spiritual level as the believer depends upon God for strength as they pray and fast from food for various reasons. Most of the leading authorities on fasting today agree that juice fasting is far superior to a water fast.

According to Dr. Rangar Berg, the world -famous biochemist and authority on nutrition, "During fasting the body burns up and excretes huge amounts of accumulated wastes". We can help this cleansing process by drinking alkaline juice instead of water while fasting. Elimination of uric acid and other inorganic acids will be accelerated. And sugars in juices will strengthen the heart, juice fasting is, therefore, the best form of fasting. Vitamins, minerals, enzymes and trace elements in fresh, raw vegetable and fruit juices are extremely beneficial in normalizing all the body processes. And as I said before, unless the fasting has been directed by the Holy Spirit and done for spiritual reasons use wisdom in all things.

Nutrients supply essential elements for the body's own healing activity and cell regeneration and thus speeding the recovery. All juices should be prepared from fresh fruit immediately before drinking. Canned or frozen juices should not be used, even though I know in some places fresh fruits are not readily available. A precautionary measure which must be observed in all cases of fasting is the complete emptying of the bowels at the beginning of the fast by getting a colonic done so that the individual is not bothered by gas or decomposing matter formed from the excrements remaining in the body.

Colon hydrotherapy sessions can be administered during the fasting period which speeds up the healing and metabolism process. The person should get as much fresh air as possible and should drink plain lukewarm water when thirsty, cold or extra hot fluids are not good for the stomach during fasting. Fresh juices may be diluted with pure water.

The total liquid intakeshould be approximately six to eight glasses. A lot of energy is spent during the fast in the process of eliminating accumulatedpoisons and toxic waste materials. It is, therefore, of utmost importance that the person gets as much physical rest and mental relaxation as possible during the fast.

In cases of fasts in which fruit juices are taken, especially when fresh grapes, oranges or grapefruit are used exclusively, the toxic wastes enter the blood - stream rapidly, resulting in an overload of toxic matter, which affects normal bodily functions. This often results in dizzy spells, followed by diarrhea and vomiting. If thisphysical reaction persists, it is advisable to discontinue the fast and take cooked vegetables containing adequate roughage such as spinach and beets until the body functioning returns to normal. The overweight person finds it much easier to go without food.

Loss of weight causes no fear and the patient's attitude makes fasting almost a pleasure. The first day's hunger pangs are perhaps the most difficult to bear. The craving for food will, however, gradually decrease as the fast progresses. Seriously sick persons have no desire for food and fasting comes naturally to them. The simples rule is to stop eating until the appetite returns naturally or until one feels completely well. Only very simple exercises like short walks may be undertaken during the fast. Awarm water or neutral bath may be taken during the period. Cold baths are not advisable. Fasting sometimes produces a state of sleeplessness which can be overcome by a warm bath, hot water bottles at the feet and by drinking one or two glasses of hot water. Those of you in the cold can appreciate this.

Chapter 8

Benefits of Fasting

There are several benefits of fasting spiritually or health wise. Did you know that during a long fast, the body feeds upon its reserves? Yes. Being deprived of needed nutrients, particularly of protein and fats, it will burn and digest its own tissues by the process of autolysis or self-digestion. "For I am fearfully and wonderfully made:" Psalms 149:14. The body will first decompose and burn those cells and tissues which are diseased, damaged, aged or dead. The essential tissues and vital organs, the glands, the nervous system and the brain are not damaged or digested in fasting. Here lies the secret of the effectiveness of fasting as a curative and rejuvenation method.

During fasting, the rebuilding of new and healthy cells starts speeded up by the amino acids released from the diseased cells. The capacity of the eliminative organs, that is, lungs, liver, kidneys, colon and the skin is greatly increased as they are relieved of the usual burden of digesting food and eliminating the waste. They are, therefore, able to quickly expel old accumulated wastes and toxins. Fasting affords a physiological rest to the digestive, assimilative and protective organs. As a result, the digestion of food and the utilization of nutrients are greatly improved after fasting. The fast also exerts a normalizing, stabilizing and rejuvenating effect on all the vital physiological, anatomical, nervous and mental functions.

The success of the fast depends largely on how it is broken. This is the most significant phase. The main rules for breaking the fast are: nothing too hot to drink, do not overeat, eat slowly and chew your food thoroughly; and take several days for the gradual change to the normal diet. If the transition to eating solid foods is carefully planned, there will be no stomach or abdominal

discomfort or damage. The individual should also continue to take rest during the transition period. The right food after a fast is as important and decisive for proper results as the fast itself. I hope you have learnt a few things thus far.

Chapter 9

Miracles of the Alkalizing Diet

The human body is composed of various organs and parts, which are made up of tissues and cells. These tissues and cells are composed of several chemical elements. The balance or equilibrium of these chemical elements in the body is an essential factor in the maintenance of health and healing of disease. The acid-alkaline balance plays a vital role in this balanced body chemistry. The pH scale is 0 = acid, 7 = neutral and 14 = alkaline.

All foods, after digestion and absorption leave either an acid or alkaline ash in the body depending on their mineral composition. The normal body chemistry is approximately 20% acid and 80% alkaline. This is the acid-alkaline balance. In normal health, the reaction of the blood is alkaline and that is essential for our physical and mental well-being. The amount of alkalis in the blood is due to the fact that the products of the vital combustions taking place in the body are mostly acid in character.

Carbohydrates and fats form about nine-tenths of the normal fuel of the body. In normal health, this great mass of material is converted into carbon dioxide gas and water. Half of the remaining one-tenth fuel is also converted into the same gas and water. This huge amount of acid is transported by the blood to the various points of discharge, mainly the lungs and also the skin (sweat) and kidneys (urine). By virtue of alkalinity, the blood is able to transport the acid from the tissues to the discharge points.

Chapter 10

The Danger of Acidosis

Whenever the alkalinity of the blood is reduced, even slightly, its ability to transport the carbon dioxide to the lungs gets reduced. This results in the accumulation of acid in the tissues. This condition is known as acidosis or hypo-alkalinity of the blood. Its symptoms are hunger, indigestion, burning sensation and pain in the pharynx, nausea, vomiting, headache, dark yellow urine, various nervous disorders and drowsiness.

Acidosis is the breeding ground for most diseases. Rheumatism, premature ageing, weight gain, arteriosclerosis, high blood pressure, skin disorders, joint pain and various degenerative diseases are traceable to this condition. Acidosis seriously interferes with the functions of the glands and organs of the body. It also lowers the vitality of the system, thereby increasing the danger of infectious diseases.

The main cause of acidosis or hypo-alkalinity of the blood is faulty diet, in which too many acid forming foods have been consumed. In the normal process of metabolism or converting the food into energy by the body, various acids are formed in the system and in addition, other acids are introduced in food.

Whenever there is substantial increase in the formation of acids in the system and these acids are not properly eliminated through the lungs, the kidneys, urine and the bowels (colon) in a timely manner, the alkalinity of the blood is reduced, resulting in acidosis. Other causes of acidosis are depletion of alkali reserve due to diarrhea, dysentery and cholera. Acidosis can be prevented by maintaining a proper balance between acid and alkaline foods in the diet and proper elimination. Certain foods leave alkaline ash and help in maintaining the alkalinity of the food, while others leave highly acid ash and lower the alkali reserve of the blood and tissue fluids to a very large extent. Eggs, coffee, sodas all do the same but are less stronger than meats. Beer, alcohol, cereals of all kinds, including all sorts of breads are also acid-forming foods, though much less than meats. All fruits, with exceptions of plums and prunes, all green and root vegetables are highly alkaline foods and help to alkalinize the blood and other tissue fluids. Beet root is an excellent blood and alkaline booster.

Thus, our daily diet should consist of mostly alkaline-forming foods such as juicy fruits, water melon, papaya, coconut water is very alkaline, also lemon, cucumber, legumes, celery, ripe fruits, leafy and root vegetables. Acid-forming foods containing concentrated proteins and starches consist of red meat, most fish, chicken, bread and cereals. Eating sensibly in this manner will ensure the necessary alkalinity of the food which will keep the body in perfect health. Whenever a person has acidosis, the higher the ratio of alkaline forming foods in the diet, is the quicker they will be the recover. Acids are always neutralized by alkaline.

An over acidic body can lead to other complications like peptic or stomach ulcers. Peptic Ulcer refers to an eroded lesion in the gastric (stomach) and intestinal mucosa. An ulcer may form in any part of the digestive tract which is exposed to acid gastric juice, but is usually found in the stomach and the duodenum (the first part of the intestines). The ulcer located in the stomach is known as gastric ulcer. Usually they are both grouped together and called peptic ulcer.

I always recommend to my clients suffering from various ailments to eat adequate alkaline foods to offset the effects of acidity and leave a safe margin of alkalinity. The most agreeable and convenient means of alkalizing the blood are citrus fruits and fruit juices. The alkalizing value of most citrus fruits, are due to large percentage of alkaline salts, mainly potash, which they contain. Each pint of organic or fresh squeezed orange juice

contains 12 grains of potassium, one of the most potent of alkalis. Lemon juice contains nine grains of the alkali to the pint and grape seven grains.

Chapter 11

Western Diets and Diseases

Foods are classified as acid-producing or alkaline-producing depending on their reaction on the urine. Calcium, magnesium, sodium and potassium present in foods contribute to the alkaline effect, while sulphur, phosphorous and chlorine contribute to the cidic effect. Depending on the pre-dominating constituents in a particular food, it is classified as acid-forming or alkaline-forming. The effect of food stuffs upon the alkalinity of the blood depends upon their residue which they leave behind after undergoing oxidation in the body. It is an error to presume that because a food tastes acidic, it has an acidic reaction in the blood.

I have learnt recently, that fruits and vegetables have organic acids in combination with soda and potash in the form of acid salts. When the acids are burnt or utilized in the body, the alkaline soda or potash is left behind. Hence the effect of the natural fruit acids is to increase the alkalinity of the blood rather than reduce it. Most drugs (especially antibiotics) are acidic, artificial chemical sweeteners like, NutraSweet, sweet 'n' low and equal all contain a poisonous substance called aspartame that is extremely acidic and can cause more harm than good to organs In the diet during any kind of disease, breakfast may consist of fresh fruits, lunch may comprise raw vegetables with acid and sub-acid fruits, and for dinner raw and cooked vegetables, or light starchy vegetables like beet, carrot, cauliflower, egg-plant and squashes may be taken.

Sweet fruits may be added to the diet after7 days. Remember, most disease casing bacteria survive in an acidic environment. Acidic Class A – Acid forming foods: barley, eggs, bananas (unripe) grain foods, beans, lentils bread, meats, cereals, nuts except almonds, cakes, oatmeal, chicken, peas, confections, (ketchup, mustard) white rice, corn, regular vinegar, sugar, chocolate, sea foods, coffee and some teas. Other Acidic Classes: Beer = pH 2.2 very acidic, Coco Cola = pH 2 extremely acidic and coffee pH = 4 Alkaline Class B – Alkaline forming foods: almonds, water melon, other melons, wheatgrass, sweet potatoes, spirulina (fresh water algae), garlic, apples, milk, green peas, broccoli, chlorella, apricots, onion, banana, (ripe) oranges, beet, parsley, cabbage, peaches, carrot, pears, cauliflower, pineapple, celery, potatoes, coconut (water and jelly), pumpkins, cottage cheese, radishes, cucumber, raisins, dates, spinach, Figs (fresh and dry) soya beans, grapes, tomatoes, lemons, turnips, lettuce and most dark green leafy vegetables.

Note: Bragg's apple cider vinegar is alkaline forming in the body. Last but not least, remember the 80/20 rule. Eat and drink 80% alkaline forming foods and 20% acid forming foods. I highly recommend you get my other health education book "The health Benefits of Coconut oil, water and jelly" if you have not done so already.

Chapter 12

Raw Juice Therapy

Raw juice therapy is a method of treatment of disease through an exclusive diet of juices of fruits and vegetables. It is also known as juice fasting. It is the most effective way to restore health and rejuvenate the body. During raw juice therapy, the eliminative and cleansing capacity of the organs of elimination, namely lungs, liver, kidneys and the skin, is greatly increased and masses of accumulated metabolic waste and toxins are quickly eliminated.

Raw juice therapy affords a physiological rest to the digestive and assimilative organs. After the juice fasting or raw juice therapy, the digestion of food and the utilization of nutrients are vastly improved. An exclusive diet of raw juices of fruits and vegetables results in much faster recovery from diseases and more effective cleansing and regeneration of the tissues than the fasting on pure water. Dr. Ragnar Berg, a world-renowned authority on nutrition and biochemistry observed:

"During fasting the body burns up and excretes huge amounts of accumulated wastes". We can help this cleansing process by drinking alkaline juices instead of water while fasting. I have done and recommended many fasts and made extensive examinations and tests and effects of fasting, and I am convinced that drinking alkali-forming fruit and vegetable juices, instead of pure water (except for spiritual related fasts), during fasting will increase the healing effect of the body. Elimination of uric acid and other inorganic acids will be accelerated. And sugars in juices will strengthen the heart. I can testify that juice fasting is, therefore, the best form of fasting for healing the body of various ailments. "As juices are extracted from plants and fruits, they process definite medicinal properties and is readily absorbed by the body and assimilated as need just as God designed it to be from day one.

Specific juices are beneficial in specific conditions. Besides specific medicinal virtues, raw fruit and vegetable juices have an extraordinary revitalizing and rejuvenating effect on all the organs, cells, tissues, glands and overall functioning of the body. The most favorable effect of raw juices in the treatment of disease is attributed to the following facts:

Raw juices of fruits and vegetables are extremely rich in vitamins, minerals, trace elements, enzymes and natural sugars. They exercise beneficial effect in normalizing all the body functions. They supply needed elements for the body's own healing activity and cell regeneration, thereby speeding the recovery process. This is great news to me.

1. The juices extracted from raw fruits and vegetables require no digestion and almost all their vital nutrients are assimilated directly in the bloodstream via the stomach and small intestine.

2. Raw juices are extremely rich in alkaline elements. This is highly beneficial in normalizing acid-alkaline balance in the blood and tissues as there is over-acidity in most conditions of ill-health.

3. Youthfulness, Generous amounts of easily absorbable organic minerals are found in raw juices especially calcium, potassium and silicon help in restoring biochemical and mineral balance in the tissues and cells, thereby preventing premature ageing of cells and disease.

4. Raw juices contain certain amount of natural medicines, vegetal hormones and antibiotics. For instance, string beans aresaid to contain insulin-like substance. Certain hormones needed by the pancreas to produce insulin are present in cucumber and onion juices. Fresh juices of garlic, onions, radish and tomatoes contain antibiotic substances.

Precautions: Just like anything else use wisdom and let everything be done in moderation. Certain precautions are necessary in adopting an exclusive diet of raw juices. Firstly, all juices should be made fresh immediately before drinking. Canned and frozen juices are processed and should be avoided as much as possible. It is advisable that one should have one's own juicer for extracting fresh juices and vegetables in its fullness. We have a Ninja Master Pre Juice Extractor and have recently bought a Nutri Bullet which is much better for smoothies.

Secondly, only fresh ripe fruits and vegetables, preferably organically grown, should be used for raw juice therapy. Thirdly, only juice the amount need for immediate consumption. Raw juices oxidizes (breaks down) rapidly and lose their medicinal value in storage, even under refrigeration.

Fourthly, the quality of the juices has a distinct bearing on the results obtained. In case of incomplete extraction of juices, their effective power is proportionately reduced due to the absence of the vitamins and enzymes which are left behind in fiber and the pulp.

Finally, if juices are too sweet they should be diluted in water on 50/50 basis or mixed with other less sweet juices. This is especially important in some specific conditions such as persons with diabetes, hypoglycemia, arthritis and high blood pressure. Fruit and vegetable juices may be divided into six main types:

(1) Juices from sweet fruits such as prunes and grapes.

(2) Juices from sub-acid fruits like apple, plum, pear, peach, apricot and cherry,

(3) Juices from acid fruits like orange, lemon, grapefruit, strawberry and pineapple.

(4) Juices from vegetable fruits, namely, tomato and cucumber.

(5) Juices from green leafy vegetables like cabbage, celery, lettuce, spinach, parsley and watercress.

(6) Juices from root vegetables like beetroot, carrot, onion, potato and radish.

In other words, fruit juices helps to stir up toxins and acids in the body, thereby stimulating the eliminative processes. Vegetable juices, on the other hand, soothe the nerves and work in a much milder manner. They carry away toxic matter in a gentle way.

Due to their differing actions fruit and vegetable juices should not be used at the same time or mixed together and I will talk about food combination at another time. It is best to use juices individually and space them for best results. In any case not more than three juices should be used in any one mixture.

The following broad rules apply when using mixtures of juices: Juices from sweet fruits may be combined with juices of sub-acid fruits, but not with those of acid fruits (too much acid at once), vegetable fruits or vegetables.

1. Juices from sub-acid fruits may be combined with juices of sweet fruits, or acid fruits, but not with other juices.

2. Juices from acid fruits may be combined with those of sub-acid fruits or vegetable fruits, but not with other juices.

3. Juices from vegetable fruits may be combined with those of acid fruits or of green leafy vegetables, but not with other juices.

4. Juices from green leafy vegetables may be combined with those of vegetable fruits or of the root vegetable, but not with other juices.

5. Juices from root vegetables may be combined with those of green leafy vegetables, but not with other juices. A proper selection of juices in treating a particular ailment is very essential. Thus, for instance, juices of carrot, cucumber, cabbage and other vegetables are very valuable in asthma, arthritis, vision problems and skin diseases.

Chapter 13

The Caribbean Juice Medley for Common Ailments

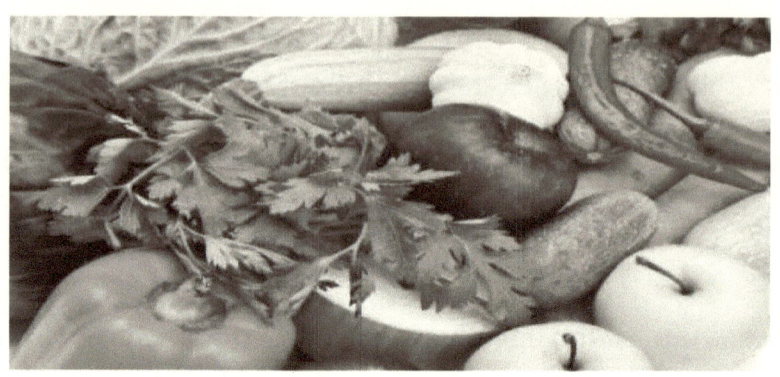

Acidity: Grapes, orange, carrot, spinach, mosambi a citrus fruit commonly used in India as (sweet lime) unlike lime it is not acidic and is said to be rich in vitamin C.

Acne: Grapes, pear, plum, tomato, cucumber, carrot, potato and spinach.

Allergies: Apricot, grapes, carrot, beet and spinach.

Arteriosclerosis: Grapefruit, pineapple, lemon, celery, carrot, lettuce, and spinach.

Anemia: Apricot, prune, strawberry, red grape, beet, celery, carrot and spinach.

Arthritis: Sour cherry, pineapple, apple, lemon, grapefruit, cucumber, beet, carrot, lettuce and spinach.

Asthma: Apricot, lemon, pineapple, peach, carrot, radish and celery.

Bronchitis: Apricot, lemon, pineapple, peach, tomato, carrot, onion and spinach.

Bladder Ailments: Apple, apricot, lemon, cucumber, carrot, celery, parsley and watercress.

Blood Pressure: Beet root, celery, carrot, cucumber, garlic, onion, aloe vera, (dash of cayenne pepper). No garlic if on blood thinning medication

Colds: Lemon, orange, grapefruit, pineapple, carrot, onion, celery and spinach.

Constipation: Apple, pear, grapes, lemon, carrot, beet, spinach and watercress.

Colitis: Apple, apricot, pear, peach, pineapple, papaya, carrot, beet, cucumber and spinach.

Diabetes: Citrus fruits, carrot, celery, lettuce and spinach.

Diarrhea: Papaya, lemon, pineapple, carrot and celery.

Eczema: Red grapes, carrot, spinach, cucumber and beet.

Epilepsy: Red grapes, figs, carrot, celery and spinach.

Eye Disorders: Apricot, tomato, carrot, celery, parsley and spinach.

Gout: Red sour cherries, pineapple, tomato, cucumber, beet, carrot, celery and spinach.

Halitosis: Apple, grapefruit, lemon, pineapple, tomato, carrot, celery and spinach.

Headache: Grapes, lemon, carrot, lettuce and spinach and plenty water.

Heart Disease: Red grapes, lemon, cucumber, carrot, beet and spinach.

High blood pressure: Grapes, orange, cucumber, carrot and beet.

Influenza: Apricot, orange, lemon, grapefruit, pineapple, carrot, onion and spinach.

Insomnia: Apple, grapes, lemon, lettuce, carrot and celery.

Jaundice: Lemon, grapes, pear, carrot, celery, spinach, beet and cucumber.

Kidney Disorders: Apple, orange, lemon, cucumber, cucumber, carrot, celery, parsley and beet.

Liver ailments: Lemon, papaya, grapes, carrot, tomato, beet and cucumber.

Menstrual Disorders: Grapes, prunes, cherry, spinach, lettuce turnips and beet.

Menopausal Symptoms: Fruits and Vegetables in season.

Neuritis: Orange, pineapple, apple, carrot and beet.

Obesity: Lemon, grapefruit, orange, cherry, pineapple, papaya, tomato, beet, cabbage, lettuce, spinach and carrot.

Piles: Lemon, orange, papaya, pineapple, carrot, spinach, turnip and watercress.

Prostate Troubles: All fruit juices in season, carrot, asparagus, lettuce and spinach.

Psoriasis: Grapes, carrot, beet, and cucumber.

Rheumatism: Grapes, orange, lemon, grapefruit, tomato, cucumber, beet, carrot and spinach.

Stomach Ulcers: Apricot, grapes, cabbage and carrots.

Sinus Trouble: Apricot, lemon, tomato, carrot, onion and radish.

Sore Throat: Apricot, grapes, lemon, pineapple, prune, tomato, carrot and parsley.

Tonsillitis: Apricot, lemon, orange, grapefruit, pineapple, carrot, spinach and radish.

Varicose Veins: Grapes, orange, plum, tomato, beetroot carrot and watercress.

Garlic: is a great natural antibiotic but it is also a natural blood thinner, use cautiously if you are taking anti-coagulant (anticlotting drugs) as prescribed by your medical doctor. Garlic is similar to aspirin which also thins the blood.

Cayenne Pepper: very good for the blood, blood pressure and for cleaning the arteries (if you can tolerate it in tea form) also very good for joint pains as a salve (don't put on open wounds) If you have stomach ulcers use cautiously.

When you decide to go on a raw juice therapy, try and drink a glass at least every three hours if you can afford it. One can thus take juices five to six times a day. A glass of water mixed with lemon juice and half of teaspoon of organic honey may be taken first thing in the morning on an empty stomach.

The raw juice diet can be continued for up to 30 days without any ill or side-effects. This is something we have done on a regular basis over the years and know that it works. Try and take adequate rest during the raw juice therapy. Raw juice acts as a cleansing agent, and starts to eliminate toxins and morbid matter from the system via the colon immediately.

Sometimes this cleansing process can result in symptoms such as pain in the abdomen (griping), diarrhea, loss of weight, headache, fever, weakness, sleeplessness and bad breath. These reactions, which are part of the cleansing process, should not be suppressed by the use of synthetic drugs. The effects will cease when the body is able to expel all toxins. After the raw juice therapy, the return to a normal balanced diet should be gradual, and in stages. Avoid very hot drinks and food right after the raw juice therapy.

Chapter 14

Constipation

Constipation is a common disturbance of the digestive tract, in this condition, the bowels (colon) do not move regularly, or are not completely emptied when they move. Constipation is the chief cause of many diseases as such a condition produces toxins which find their way into the blood stream through the wall of the colon and are carried to all parts of the body. This results in weakening of the vital organs and lowering of the resistance of the entire system. Appendicitis, rheumatism, arthritis, high blood pressure, diabetes, multiple sclerosis, lupus, cataract and even cancer are only a few of the diseases in which chronic constipation is an important predisposing factor.

The number of motions required for normal health varies from person to person. Most people have one motion or bowel movement per day, some have two or three while others have one every other day or week. However, for comfort and health, at least one clear bowel movement a day is important, but two or three should be your goal. Pay more attention to your bowel movements

The most common symptoms of constipation are infrequency, irregularity or difficulty of elimination due to hard (impacted) fecal matter. Among the other symptoms are a coated tongue, foul breath, loss of appetite, headache, dizziness, dark circles under the eyes, depression, nausea, pimples on the face, ulcer in the mouth, burning stomach, constant fullness in the abdomen due to bloating, in some instances diarrhea alternating with constipation, varicose veins, pain in the lumber (lower back) region, acidity, heart burn, irritability, fatigue, insomnia (sleeplessness) and overall low feeling.

The Colon

Your whole circulatory system is locked
into the the colon

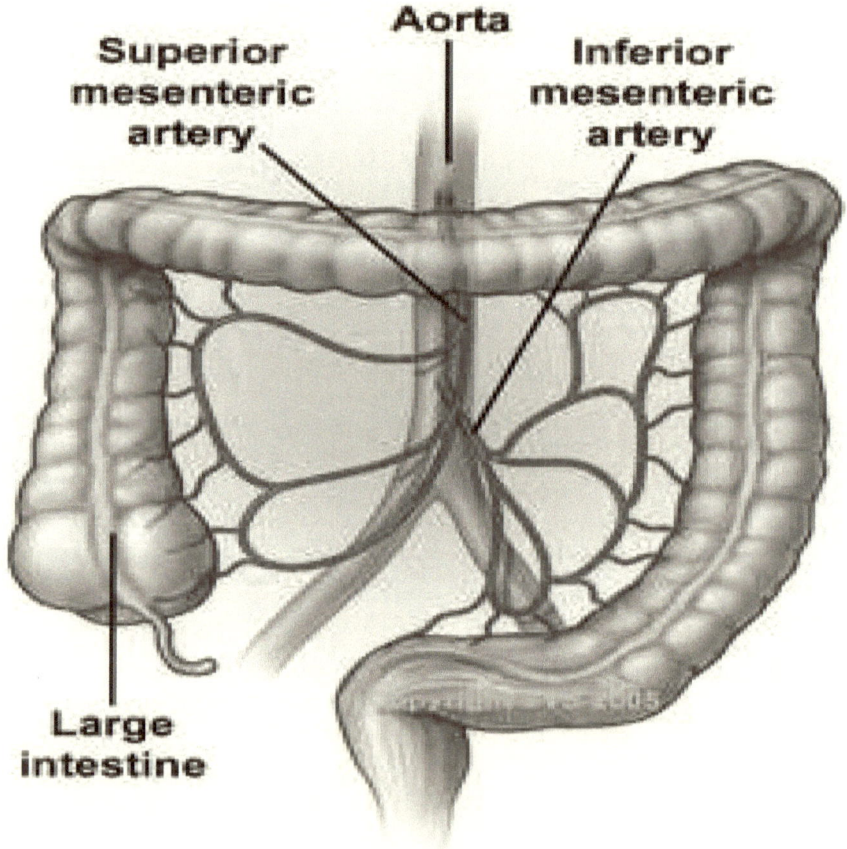

Chapter 15

Testimonies

In my practice as a naturopathic practitioner and clinical colon therapist, I have seen several children between the ages of 9 and 14 years who were severely constipated. Here are just a few testimonies about the benefits of colon therapy.

Testimony: I can remember a mother bringing her 11 year old daughter who was crying and in pain, because she didn't use the bathroom for almost two weeks. After a consultation I gave her a colonic using the proper techniques and timing for children, and when she was through she almost hugged the wind out of me.

Testimony: A young man come in with his mother who looked so worried, he was suffering from candidiasis in his mouth which had turned into a painful mouth ulcer. His mouth and tongue was covered in a thick white coating, he had lost weight because he couldn't eat. His mother said she had taken him to several doctors who prescribed antibiotics, but instead of getting better he kept getting worst by now he could only suck fluid through a straw on one side of his jaw. I proceeded with a colonic and recommended one colonic for three weeks and omitted all sugar.

Two days after the colonic the mother called to say her son's tongue was clearing up and turning pink again. By the second session he was eating food and full of smile, and by the third session his mouth ulcer was gone, his mouth and tongue was cleared of the thick white coating and he was able to return to school after missing out so many classes. They were both happy.

Testimony: Another lady was brought in by her sister who was diagnosed with lupus and was very constipated, she also had a heart condition. I contacted her cardiologist to inform him that his patient had come in for a colonic and if he had any objections. He was most pleased to see me contact him prior to doing the colonic and after explaining my experience and qualifications he gave the approval and asked I give him a report after, which I did. After doing my routine health checks and consultation I realized the client was also suffering from candida overgrowth (chronic yeast infection) after the first colon therapy session the client was more alert, the white coating on her tongue had already started to clear, and by the second session her tongue was pink and she was happy and said her appetite had returned and she was eating. Few weeks after her she called to say she was up and about and had returned to work.

Testimoy: A young lady came in complaining of having bouts of yeast infections, and said she has been having this problem for some time. I recommend she do three colon therapy sessions in three weeks and exclude all sugar. Sure enough for months she said she had no yeast infection problem.

Testimony: A gentleman in his late 60's who was to have a barium enema, prior to colonoscopy was referred to us by one of the local diagnostic centers for a ColoLavage (colon therapy / colonoscopy type prep) after they failed to see the walls of his large intestine due to impacted feces. The client said he was vomiting and felt sick after drinking what he was told to drink and did not complete it. After the session he proceeded to his doctor's office to have his procedure done. I later called the doctor for a rating of the ColoLavage and she was very pleased and said the colon was 85-95% cleansed. This was my big break! They continue to send clients to me until this day. I could go on with testimonies about clients with drug addictions, multiple sclerosis, yeast infections, bloating, back pain, fatigue etc. Who have benefited from colon therapy.

Apart from the colonics I also recommended prebiotics and a good strain of probiotics, eliminate all sugar (including in fruits) and some other advice of which you will hear when you come and see me or in my other books. Due to the western diet, which mainly consist of GMO's – genetically modified organism, which in truth is not real food but is all artificial, the body has a hard time digesting and absorbing this kind of stuff. And this is what our children are being fed on 24/7 at home and in our schools, no wonder they are constipated, sick, hyper active and have learning problems.

Chapter 16

Cause of Most Constipation

The most important causes for chronic constipation are wrong diet and a faulty style of living. All foods in their natural state contain a good percentage of 'roughage, fiber' which is most essential in preserving natural balance of foods and also in helping peristalsis - the natural rhythmic action of the bowels by means of which the food is passed down the alimentary canal. Much of the food we eat today is genetically modifies organisms (GMO) processed, packed with sodium (salt) and is very deficient in natural bulk or roughage and this results in chronic constipation.

Intake of refined and rich food lacking in vitamins and minerals, insufficient intake of water, consumption of meat in large quantities, excessive use of bush teas (including herbal teas) coffee, insufficient chewing, late night snacking, overeating, wrong combination of foods, irregular habits of eating and drinking may all contribute to poor bowel function. Other causes include faulty and irregular habit of defecation, frequent use of purgatives (laxatives), weakness of abdominal muscles due to sedentary habits, lack of physical activity and emotional stress and strain. Ignoring going to the bathroom, when nature calls is also very dangerous to your health.

Diseases such as tumors or growths, a sluggish liver, colitis, spastic condition of the intestine, diverticulosis, hyperacidity, diseases of the rectum and colon, bad teeth, uterine diseases, diabetes, stroke, smoking, use of certain drugs for treating other ailments, abnormal condition of the lower spine and enlargement of the prostate glands, pregnancy and certain medication can also cause chronic constipation.

The most important factor in solving constipation is a natural and simple diet and a series of colonics (colon therapy, colon irrigation) to rid the entire length of the colon (ascending, transverse and descending colon) of impacted feces.

Before you say yes, remember you have a right to know the qualification, training, certification and experience of anyone who is touching your body or going to treat you. Your diet should consist of unrefined food such as whole grain cereals, bran, honey, molasses, and lentils; green and leafy vegetables, especially spinach, string beans, tomatoes, lettuce, onion, cabbage, cauliflower, sprouts, celery, turnip, pumpkin, peas, beetroot, asparagus, carrot; fresh fruits, especially watermelon, pears, grapes, papayas, mangoes, grapefruit, berries, guava and oranges etc.

The diet alone is not enough. Food should be properly chewed-each morsel for at least 15 times. Hurried meals and meals at odd times should be avoided. Sugar and sugary foods should be strictly avoided because sugar steals B vitamins from the body, without which the intestines cannot function normally. Foods which constipate are all products made of white flour, white rice, bread, cakes, pastries, biscuits, cheese, fleshy foods, preservatives, and white sugar. Again I will say, let everything be done in moderation.

Chapter 17

Water and Constipation

Regular drinking of purified, distilled water is beneficial not only for constipation and rehydration, but also for cleaning the entire system, diluting the blood, washing out toxins and poisonous substances. The human body is made up of 75% - 80% distilled water. Normally 6-8 glasses of water should be taken daily as it is essential for digesting and dissolving food particles and nutrients so that they can be readily absorbed by the body. The small intestines, absorbs water and nutrients and large intestine or colon absorbs water and electrolytes. As stated in my book "The Health Benefits of Coconut Oil, Water and Jelly" coconut water is a natural diuretic.

The ratio of friendly and pathogenic bacteria in the gut is 80% good or friendly bacteria to 20% pathogenic or bad bacteria. Majority of persons is suffering from microbial imbalance (dysbiosis) in the gut. Contrary to the myths that colon therapy washes out the good bacteria (flora) majority of the population has more bad bacteria than good.

Water and cold drinks should not be taken with meals as it dilutes the gastric juices essential for proper digestion in the stomach. Water should be taken either half an hour before or an hour after meals. Generally all fruits, except banana and jackfruit, are beneficial in the treatment of constipation. Certain fruits are however more effective.

Avocado pears are regarded the as one of the best fruit beneficial in the treatment of constipation. Avocados are a good source of potassium, vitamin C, B and K, fiber and the good fat found in this fruit helps to lubricate the colon. Patients suffering from chronic constipation should better adopt an exclusive diet of this fruit for few days, but in ordinary cases a slice taken with meals will have the desired effect.

The same is true of guava which, when eaten with seeds, gives roughage to the diet and helps in the normal evacuation of the bowels. Grapes and prunes have also proved highly beneficial in overcoming constipation. The combination of the properties of the cellulose, sugar and organic acid in grapes and prunes make them a laxative food. Their field of action is not limited to clearing the bowels only. They also tone up the stomach and intestines and relieve the most chronic constipation. When fresh grapes or prunes are not available, raisins soaked in water can be used.

Raisins should be soaked in a glass of drinking water for 24 to 48 hours. This would swell them to the original size of the grapes. The raisins should be eaten early in the morning. The water in which raisins are soaked should be drunk along with the soaked raisins.

I understand, drinking hot water with lemon or lime juice and half a teaspoon of salt is also an effective remedy for constipation. If you have high blood, pressure doesn't do this because salt retains water in the body. Drinking water which has been kept overnight in a copper vessel, the first thing in the morning will bring good results. Also understand that linseed is extremely useful in difficult cases of constipation. A teaspoon of linseed swallowed with water before each meal provides both bulk and lubrication.

In all ordinary cases of severe constipation, an exclusive fruit diet for about seven days would be the best way to begin the treatment. For long-standing and stubborn cases, it should be advisable to have a short fast for four or five days followed by a series of colon therapy. This will remove the packed contents of the bowels, eliminate toxins and purify the blood stream. Weak and sick patients should always consult with their medical doctor before partaking in any form of dieting.

What next?
After the all-fruit diet or the short fast, as the case may be, the person should gradually embark upon a balanced diet comprising adequate raw foods, ripe fruits and whole grain cereals. The bowels should be cleansed regularly with warm filtered purified water which is what most certified colon therapists are trained to use. Colon hydrotherapy is one of the best treatments one can have done prior, during and after any kind of illness including chemotherapy and radiation treatments. Colonics helps to rid the body of drug sediments that might be in the feces in the colon and transferred into the blood stream. I will discuss this in another book.

Depending on where you are living, an alternate hot and cold hip bath taken before retiring to bed is also beneficial. Abdominal exercise and manual or mechanical vibratory massage have a refreshing and stimulating effect in many cases. Exercise plays a vital role in strengthening and activating the muscles, thereby preventing constipation.

Chapter 18

Fatigue

Fatigue refers to a feeling of tiredness or weariness. It can be temporary or chronic. Almost every person has to work overtime on certain occasions, sacrificing rest and sleep, which may cause temporary fatigue. This condition can be remedied by adequate rest. Chronic or continuous fatigue is, however, a serious problem which requires a comprehensive plan of treatment. Chronic fatigue can result from a variety of factors. A specific character trait, compulsiveness, worrying, unforgiveness, and negative thinking can lead to continuous fatigue. Many persons constantly feel that they cannot take rest until they finish everything that needs to be done at one time in one day. These persons are usually perfectionists, tense and cannot relax unless they complete the whole job, no matter how tired they may be.

The chief cause of fatigue is lowered vitality or lack of energy due to wrong feeding habits. Fatigue is an indication that the cells of the body are not getting sufficient live atoms and nutrients in the food to furnish them with a constant flow of needed energy. The habitual use of refined processed foods such as white sugar, refined cereals and white four products as well as processed and preserved foods have a very bad effect on the system in general.

Foods in this way are deprived, to a very great extent, of their invaluable vitamins and minerals. Such foods lead to nervousness, tiredness, obesity and a host of other complaints prevalent today. Certain physical conditions can cause fatigue. Anemia (low blood count) is a very common ailment leading to tiredness. It is known as 'tired blood' disturbance. In anemia, very little oxygen reaches the tissues with the result energy cannot be produced normally.

This causes constant tiredness and mental depression. Anemia usually results from deficiencies of iron and vitamin B12. Sometime deficiencies of vitamin B6 and folic acid are also involved. Insomnia or lack of sleep can be a cause of torturing fatigue.

Sleep induced by sleeping pills and other drugs does not get rid of fatigue. Intestinal parasites can also lead to fatigue as they rob the body of good nourishment and feed themselves on rich red blood. Other ailments which can cause fatigue are low blood pressure, low blood sugar, any kind of infection in the body, liver damage, a sluggish thyroid, allergies in foods and drugs caused by additives including artificial flavors, MSG, colors and preservatives.

Mental and emotional tension is one of the major causes of fatigue. A person who is tense and cannot relax has all the muscles of his body more or less contracted. This leads to needless waste of unusually large amounts of energy. Food is continuously being burnt; lactic acid accumulates more rapidly than it can be carried to liver for conversion to body starch. Persons who are hyper, nervous, anxious, stressful and irritable usually suffer from this type of fatigue. You will keep in perfect peace those whose minds are steadfast, because they trust in you. Isaiah 26:3

Nutritional measures are most vital in the treatment of fatigue. Studies reveal that people who eat small mid-meals suffer less from fatigue and nervousness, think more clearly and are more efficient than those who eat only three meals daily. These mid-meals should consist of fresh fruit or vegetable juices, raw vegetables or small sandwich of whole grain bread. The mid-meal should be small and less food should be consumed at regular meals. Sick persons should eat healthy foods which supply energy to the body as often as possible. It is said that "Any seed or root vegetable that will grow again will renew human vitality." Persons should supplement health-building food groups with special protective foods such as milk, high quality cold-pressed unrefined coconut oil and honey. The person should also take prebiotics, probiotics, vitamins and mineral supplements as an effective assurance against nutritional deficiencies, as such deficiencies have been found to be a factor in fatigue.

Lack of pantothenic acid, B vitamin in particular, leads to extreme fatigue as deficiency of this vitamin is associated with exhaustion of the adrenal glands. In fact the entire B-complex group protects the nerves and increases energy by helping to nourish and regulate glands. I always recommend super B-complex (foods and vitamins) to my clients as these are readily found in most supermarkets. The food groups rich in vitamin B are wheat, other whole grain cereals, green leafy vegetables, milk, nuts, banana, yeast and peas. Minerals are also important. Potassium is especially needed for protection against fatigue. Raw green vegetables are rich in this mineral.

Calcium is essential for relaxation and is beneficial in cases of insomnia (sleeplessness) and tension both of which can lead to fatigue. Sodium and zinc are also beneficial in the treatment of fatigue. Raw fresh vegetable juices especially carrot juice, taken separately or in combination with beets and cucumbers, is highly valuable in overcoming fatigue.

A great combination of juices for fatigue is half glass of carrot mixed with beet and cucumber. Individuals should never seek to get a "quick fix" energy lift, by taking drugs, drinking coffee, energy drinks (red bull, monster), 5 hour energy, alcohol or eating sugar or sweets. They only give a temporary boost and this is soon followed by a serious downward plunge of energy, leaving the person feeing worse than before. This is one of the biggest mistakes persons working on night shift, school teachers, and university and college students make during times of fatigue.

About the Author

Bishop Dr. Juliette D. Fagan, Prof. A native born Caymanian, married to Pastor Leeroy Fagan. She is the owner and CEO of Healthy Solutions Colon Therapy and Detoxification Centre located in Jamaica and Grand Cayman. Dr. Fagan as she is affectionately called is a trained Practical Nurse, Cayman Islands School of Nursing, and Ex-Police Officer with The Royal Cayman Islands Police Force. She is also a gospel recording artist with two albums.

She studied Surgical Technology at Lindsey Hopkins Technical Miami Fla, Naturopathic Practitioner and Consultant at the Alternative Medicine of College of Canada, Colon Hydrotherapy, The International School for Colon Therapy USA, Clinical Colon Hydrotherapy, GI Doctors, Garden City NY with Amy Sanders of GPACT, she is Caribbean Ambassador of Global Professional Association for Colon Therapists.

She is a certified Prepare & Enrichment Family and Marital Counsellor Fla, Marriage officer Cayman Islands Government Bishop Dr. Fagan is the founder and President of Vision Miracle Churches of God Evangelistic Association and Vision Dominion School of Theology. A Graduate of the International Seminary USA, Professor of Theology, Christ Kingdom University Cameroon Africa. Radio and TV personality, author, inspirational, columnist and healthy life styles Speaker.

Conclusion:

Thus, through a faulty diet and poor elimination of waste it is not the digestive system alone which is adversely affected. When toxins accumulate, other organs such as the bowels, kidneys, skin and lungs are overworked and cannot get rid of these harmful substances as quickly as they are produced. Besides this, mental and emotional disturbances cause imbalances of the human electric field within which cell metabolism takes place, producing toxins. When the cellular level is undisturbed and nourished disease-causing germs can live in it without multiplying or producing toxins. It is only when it is disturbed or when the blood is polluted with too much acid and toxic waste that the germs multiply and become harmful.

I am not a professional writer but I have a desire to empower and educate all who are willing to learn and make adjustments in their daily walks of life. I know that as I practice I will become more perfect. Thanks for your patience and understanding and I pray you have learnt something from what I have written in this and my other books. More great books are coming out soon on inspiration, family issues, diseases, colon therapy, marriage, finances and entrepreneurship. I trust you got my first e-book or paperback on The Health Benefits of Coconut Oil, Water & Jelly and irritable bowel syndrome. My own line of natural health products coming soon!

Copy Rights

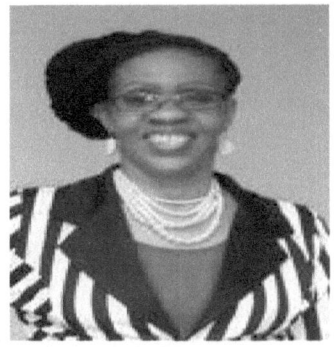

Bishop Dr Juliette D. Fagan

Email: healthy_solutions@yahoo.com
www.healthysolutionsbiz.com
www.visionmiraclecog.

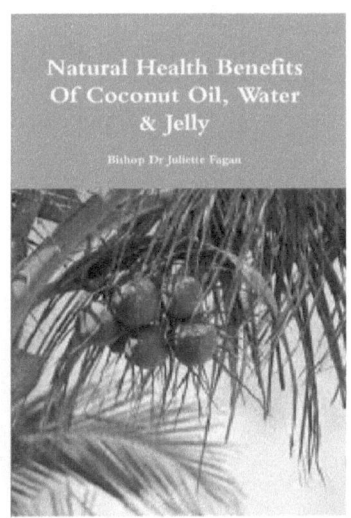

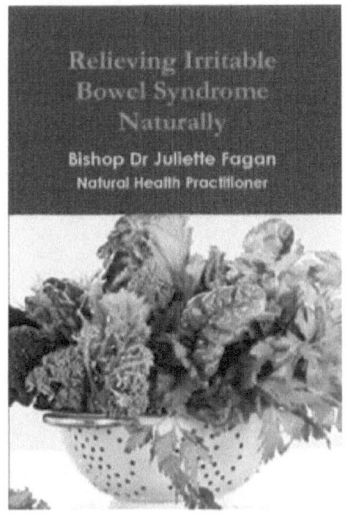

ISBN 978-1-312-04775-4

90000

9 781312 047754